HORMONE RESET DIET

MAIN COURSE - 60+ Breakfast, Lunch, Dinner and Dessert Recipes for Hormone Reset Diet

TABLE OF CONTENTS

purposes solely, and is universal as so. The presentation of the information is without contract or any type of guarantee assurance.

The trademarks that are used are without any consent, and the publication of the trademark is without permission or backing by the trademark owner. All trademarks and brands within this book are for clarifying purposes only and are the owned by the owners themselves, not affiliated with this document.

Introduction

Hormone reset recipes for personal enjoyment but also for family enjoyment. You will love them for sure for how easy it is to prepare them.

BLUEBERRY PANCAKES

Serves: *4*

Prep Time: *10*   Minutes

Cook Time: *20*   Minutes

Total Time: *30*   Minutes

INGREDIENTS

- 1 cup whole wheat flour
- ¼ tsp baking soda
- ¼ tsp baking powder
- 1 cup blueberries
- 2 eggs
- 1 cup milk

DIRECTIONS

1. In a bowl combine all ingredients together and mix well
2. In a skillet heat olive oil

3. Pour ¼ of the batter and cook each pancake for 1-2 minutes per side

4. When ready remove from heat and serve

MULBERRIES PANCAKES

Serves: **4**

Prep Time: **10**   Minutes

Cook Time: **30**   Minutes

Total Time: **40**   Minutes

INGREDIENTS

- 1 cup whole wheat flour
- ¼ tsp baking soda
- ¼ tsp baking powder
- 1 cup mulberries
- 2 eggs
- 1 cup milk

DIRECTIONS

1. In a bowl combine all ingredients together and mix well
2. In a skillet heat olive oil
3. Pour ¼ of the batter and cook each pancake for 1-2 minutes per side
4. When ready remove from heat and serve

Serves: *4*

Prep Time: *10*   Minutes

Cook Time: *20*   Minutes

Total Time: *30*   Minutes

INGREDIENTS

- 1 cup whole wheat flour
- ¼ tsp baking soda
- ¼ tsp baking powder
- 1 cup mashed banana
- 2 eggs
- 1 cup milk

DIRECTIONS

1. In a bowl combine all ingredients together and mix well
2. In a skillet heat olive oil
3. Pour ¼ of the batter and cook each pancake for 1-2 minutes per side
4. When ready remove from heat and serve

NECTARINE PANCAKES

Serves: *4*

Prep Time: *10* Minutes

Cook Time: *20* Minutes

Total Time: *30* Minutes

INGREDIENTS

- 1 cup whole wheat flour
- ¼ tsp baking soda
- ¼ tsp baking powder
- 1 cup nectarines
- 2 eggs
- 1 cup milk

DIRECTIONS

1. In a bowl combine all ingredients together and mix well
2. In a skillet heat olive oil
3. Pour ¼ of the batter and cook each pancake for 1-2 minutes per side
4. When ready remove from heat and serve

Serves: **4**
Prep Time: **10** Minutes
Cook Time: **30** Minutes
Total Time: **40** Minutes

INGREDIENTS

- 1 cup whole wheat flour
- ¼ tsp baking soda
- ¼ tsp baking powder
- 2 eggs
- 1 cup milk

DIRECTIONS

1. In a bowl combine all ingredients together and mix well
2. In a skillet heat olive oil
3. Pour ¼ of the batter and cook each pancake for 1-2 minutes per side
4. When ready remove from heat and serve

Serves: **8-12**
Prep Time: **10**   Minutes

Cook Time: **20**   Minutes

Total Time: **30**   Minutes

INGREDIENTS

- 2 eggs
- 1 tablespoon olive oil
- 1 cup milk
- 2 cups whole wheat flour
- 1 tsp baking soda
- ¼ tsp baking soda
- 1 cup peaches
- 1 tsp cinnamon
- ¼ cup molasses

DIRECTIONS

1. In a bowl combine all dry ingredients
2. In another bowl combine all dry ingredients

3. Combine wet and dry ingredients together
4. Pour mixture into 8-12 prepared muffin cups, fill 2/3 of the cups
5. Bake for 18-20 minutes at 375 F
6. When ready remove from the oven and serve

Serves: **8-12**
Prep Time: **10**   Minutes

Cook Time: **20**   Minutes

Total Time: **30**   Minutes

INGREDIENTS

- 2 eggs
- 1 tablespoon olive oil
- 1 cup milk
- 2 cups whole wheat flour
- 1 tsp baking soda
- ¼ tsp baking soda
- 1 tsp cinnamon
- 1 cup lemon slices

DIRECTIONS

1. In a bowl combine all dry ingredients
2. In another bowl combine all dry ingredients
3. Combine wet and dry ingredients together

4. Pour mixture into 8-12 prepared muffin cups, fill 2/3 of the cups

5. Bake for 18-20 minutes at 375 F

6. When ready remove from the oven and serve

Serves: **8-12**

Prep Time: **10** Minutes

Cook Time: **20** Minutes

Total Time: **30** Minutes

INGREDIENTS

- 2 eggs
- 1 tablespoon olive oil
- 1 cup milk
- 2 cups whole wheat flour
- 1 tsp baking soda
- ¼ tsp baking soda
- 1 tsp cinnamon
- 1 cup blueberries

DIRECTIONS

1. In a bowl combine all dry ingredients
2. In another bowl combine all dry ingredients
3. Combine wet and dry ingredients together

4. Fold in blueberries and mix well

5. Pour mixture into 8-12 prepared muffin cups, fill 2/3 of the cups

6. Bake for 18-20 minutes at 375 F

7. When ready remove from the oven and serve

Serves: **8-12**
Prep Time: **10**   Minutes

Cook Time: **20**   Minutes

Total Time: **30**   Minutes

INGREDIENTS

- 2 eggs
- 1 tablespoon olive oil
- 1 cup milk
- 2 cups whole wheat flour
- 1 tsp baking soda
- ¼ tsp baking soda
- 1 tsp cinnamon
- 1 cup kumquat

DIRECTIONS

1. In a bowl combine all dry ingredients
2. In another bowl combine all dry ingredients
3. Combine wet and dry ingredients together

4. Pour mixture into 8-12 prepared muffin cups, fill 2/3 of the cups

5. Bake for 18-20 minutes at 375 F

6. When ready remove from the oven and serve

Serves: *8-12*
Prep Time: *10*   Minutes

Cook Time: *20*   Minutes

Total Time: *30*   Minutes

INGREDIENTS

- 2 eggs
- 1 tablespoon olive oil
- 1 cup milk
- 2 cups whole wheat flour
- 1 tsp baking soda
- ¼ tsp baking soda
- 1 tsp cinnamon
- 1 cup chocolate chips

DIRECTIONS

1. In a bowl combine all dry ingredients
2. In another bowl combine all dry ingredients
3. Combine wet and dry ingredients together

4. Fold in chocolate chips and mix well
5. Pour mixture into 8-12 prepared muffin cups, fill 2/3 of the cups
6. Bake for 18-20 minutes at 375 F
7. When ready remove from the oven and serve

Serves: **8-12**
Prep Time: **10**   Minutes

Cook Time: **20**   Minutes

Total Time: **30**   Minutes

INGREDIENTS

- 2 eggs
- 1 tablespoon olive oil
- 1 cup milk
- 2 cups whole wheat flour
- 1 tsp baking soda
- ¼ tsp baking soda
- 1 tsp cinnamon

DIRECTIONS

1. In a bowl combine all dry ingredients
2. In another bowl combine all dry ingredients
3. Combine wet and dry ingredients together

4. Pour mixture into 8-12 prepared muffin cups, fill 2/3 of the cups

5. Bake for 18-20 minutes at 375 F

6. When ready remove from the oven and serve

Serves: *1*
Prep Time: 5   Minutes

Cook Time: *10* Minutes

Total Time: *15* Minutes

INGREDIENTS

- 2 eggs
- ¼ tsp salt
- ¼ tsp black pepper
- 1 tablespoon olive oil
- ¼ cup cheese
- ¼ tsp basil

DIRECTIONS

1. In a bowl combine all ingredients together and mix well
2. In a skillet heat olive oil and pour the egg mixture
3. Cook for 1-2 minutes per side

4. When ready remove omelette from the skillet and
   serve

Serves: **1**

Prep Time: **5** Minutes

Cook Time: **10** Minutes

Total Time: **15** Minutes

INGREDIENTS

- 2 eggs
- ¼ tsp salt
- ¼ tsp black pepper
- 1 tablespoon olive oil
- ¼ cup cheese
- ¼ tsp basil
- 1 cup carrot

DIRECTIONS

1. In a bowl combine all ingredients together and mix well
2. In a skillet heat olive oil and pour the egg mixture
3. Cook for 1-2 minutes per side

4. When ready remove omelette from the skillet and
   serve

Serves: *1*
Prep Time: *5*   Minutes

Cook Time: *10*   Minutes

Total Time: *15*   Minutes

INGREDIENTS

- 2 eggs
- ¼ tsp salt
- ¼ tsp black pepper
- 1 tablespoon olive oil
- ¼ cup cheese
- ¼ tsp basil
- 1 cup red onion

DIRECTIONS

1. In a bowl combine all ingredients together and mix well
2. In a skillet heat olive oil and pour the egg mixture
3. Cook for 1-2 minutes per side

4. When ready remove omelette from the skillet and serve

Serves: *1*

Prep Time: *5*   Minutes

Cook Time: *10*   Minutes

Total Time: *15*   Minutes

INGREDIENTS

- 2 eggs
- ¼ tsp salt
- ¼ tsp black pepper
- 1 tablespoon olive oil
- ¼ cup cheese
- ¼ tsp basil
- 1 cup broccoli

DIRECTIONS

1. In a bowl combine all ingredients together and mix well
2. In a skillet heat olive oil and pour the egg mixture
3. Cook for 1-2 minutes per side

4. When ready remove omelette from the skillet and serve

BEETS OMELETTE

Serves: **1**

Prep Time: **5**   Minutes

Cook Time: **10**   Minutes

Total Time: **15**   Minutes

INGREDIENTS

- 2 eggs
- ¼ tsp salt
- ¼ tsp black pepper
- 1 tablespoon olive oil
- ¼ cup cheese
- ¼ tsp basil
- 1 cup beets

DIRECTIONS

1. In a bowl combine all ingredients together and mix well
2. In a skillet heat olive oil and pour the egg mixture
3. Cook for 1-2 minutes per side

4. When ready remove omelette from the skillet and serve

Serves: **6-8**
Prep Time: **10**   Minutes

Cook Time: **25**   Minutes

Total Time: **35**   Minutes

INGREDIENTS

- 1 eggplant
- 12 oz. ricotta cheese
- 2 oz. mozzarella cheese
- 1 can tomatoes
- ¼ tsp salt
- 2 tablespoons seasoning

DIRECTIONS

1. Lay the eggplant on a baking sheet
2. Roast at 350 F for 12-15 minutes
3. In a bowl combine mozzarella, seasoning, tomatoes, ricotta cheese and salt
4. Add cheese mixture to the eggplant and roll

5. Place the rolls into a baking dish and bake for another 10-12 minutes

6. When ready remove from the oven and serve

Serves: **4-6**

Prep Time: **10** Minutes

Cook Time: **25** Minutes

Total Time: **35** Minutes

INGREDIENTS

- 1 lb. asparagus
- 4-5 pieces prosciutto
- ¼ tsp salt
- 2 eggs

DIRECTIONS

1. Trim the asparagus and season with salt
2. Wrap each asparagus pieces with prosciutto
3. Place the wrapped asparagus in a baking dish
4. Bake at 375 F for 22-25 minutes
5. When ready remove from the oven and serve

Serves: *8*
Prep Time: *10*   Minutes

Cook Time: *20*   Minutes

Total Time: *30*   Minutes

INGREDIENTS

- 8 eggs
- ½ cup Greek Yogurt
- 1 tablespoon mustard
- 1 tsp smoked paprika
- 1 tablespoon green onions

DIRECTIONS

1. In a saucepan add the eggs and bring to a boil
2. Cover and boil for 10-15 minutes
3. When ready slice the eggs in half and remove the yolks
4. In a bowl combine remaining ingredients and mix well
5. Spoon 1 tablespoon of the mixture into each egg

6. Garnish with green onions and serve

Serves: **6-8**
Prep Time: **5**   Minutes

Cook Time: **15**   Minutes

Total Time: **20**   Minutes

INGREDIENTS

- 2 cucumbers
- 1 cup Greek yogurt
- 1 garlic clove
- 1 tsp paprika
- 1 tsp dill
- 1 tsp chili powder

DIRECTIONS

1. In a bowl combine all ingredients together except cucumbers
2. Cut the cucumbers into rounds and scoot out the inside
3. Fill each cucumber with the spicy mixture
4. When ready sprinkle paprika and serve

SIMPLE PIZZA RECIPE

Serves: *6-8*

Prep Time: *10*   Minutes

Cook Time: *15*   Minutes

Total Time: *25*   Minutes

INGREDIENTS

- 1 pizza crust
- ½ cup tomato sauce
- ¼ black pepper
- 1 cup pepperoni slices
- 1 cup mozzarella cheese
- 1 cup olives

DIRECTIONS

1. Spread tomato sauce on the pizza crust
2. Place all the toppings on the pizza crust
3. Bake the pizza at 425 F for 12-15 minutes

4. When ready remove pizza from the oven and serve

Serves: *6-8*

Prep Time: *10*   Minutes

Cook Time: *15*   Minutes

Total Time: *25*   Minutes

INGREDIENTS

- 1 pizza crust
- ½ cup tomato sauce
- ¼ black pepper
- 1 cup zucchini slices
- 1 cup mozzarella cheese
- 1 cup olives

DIRECTIONS

1. Spread tomato sauce on the pizza crust
2. Place all the toppings on the pizza crust
3. Bake the pizza at 425 F for 12-15 minutes
4. When ready remove pizza from the oven and serve

Serves: **2**

Prep Time: **10**   Minutes

Cook Time: **20**   Minutes

Total Time: **30**   Minutes

INGREDIENTS

- ½ lb. asparagus
- 1 tablespoon olive oil
- ½ red onion
- 2 eggs
- ¼ tsp salt
- 2 oz. cheddar cheese
- 1 garlic clove
- ¼ tsp dill

DIRECTIONS

1. Boil the asparagus until tender and set aside
2. In a bowl whisk eggs with salt and cheese

3. In a frying pan heat olive oil and pour egg mixture
4. Add remaining ingredients and mix well
5. When ready serve with asparagus

Serves: *2*

Prep Time: *10*   Minutes

Cook Time: *20*   Minutes

Total Time: *30*   Minutes

INGREDIENTS

- ½ lb. red cabbage
- 1 tablespoon olive oil
- ½ red onion
- 2 eggs
- ¼ tsp salt
- 2 oz. cheddar cheese
- 1 garlic clove
- ¼ tsp dill

DIRECTIONS

1. In a bowl whisk eggs with salt and cheese
2. In a frying pan heat olive oil and pour egg mixture

3. Add remaining ingredients and mix well
4. Serve when ready

Serves: **2**

Prep Time: **10**   Minutes

Cook Time: **20**   Minutes

Total Time: **30**   Minutes

INGREDIENTS

- 1 cup kale
- 1 tablespoon olive oil
- ½ red onion
- ¼ tsp salt
- 2 eggs
- 2 oz. cheddar cheese
- 1 garlic clove
- ¼ tsp dill

DIRECTIONS

1. In a skillet sauté kale until tender
2. In a bowl whisk eggs with salt and cheese

3. In a frying pan heat olive oil and pour egg mixture

4. Add remaining ingredients and mix well

5. When ready serve with sautéed kale

Serves: **2**

Prep Time: **10** Minutes

Cook Time: **20** Minutes

Total Time: **30** Minutes

INGREDIENTS

- 1 cup brussel sprouts
- 1 tablespoon olive oil
- ½ red onion
- ¼ tsp salt
- 2 eggs
- 2 oz. parmesan cheese
- 1 garlic clove
- ¼ tsp dill

DIRECTIONS

1. In a bowl whisk eggs with salt and cheese
2. In a frying pan heat olive oil and pour egg mixture

3. Add remaining ingredients and mix well
4. Serve when ready

Serves: **2**

Prep Time: **10** Minutes

Cook Time: **20** Minutes

Total Time: **30** Minutes

INGREDIENTS

- 1 cup broccoli
- 1 tablespoon olive oil
- ½ red onion
- ¼ tsp salt
- 2 eggs
- 2 oz. cheddar cheese
- 1 garlic clove
- ¼ tsp dill

DIRECTIONS

1. In a skillet sauté broccoli until tender
2. In a bowl whisk eggs with salt and cheese

3. In a frying pan heat olive oil and pour egg mixture

4. Add remaining ingredients and mix well

5. When ready serve with sautéed broccoli

Serves: 2
Prep Time: 5   Minutes

Cook Time: 15   Minutes

Total Time: 20   Minutes

INGREDIENTS

- 1 spaghetti squash

DIRECTIONS

1. Cut the spaghetti squash in half and remove seeds
2. Spiralize the squash and set aside
3. Fill a container with water and place the squash side down in a container
4. Microwave for 5-6 minutes
5. Serve when ready

SPICY MUSSELS

Serves: **4**
Prep Time: **10** Minutes

Cook Time: **20** Minutes

Total Time: **30** Minutes

INGREDIENTS

- 2 shallots
- 2 garlic cloves
- 2 tablespoons chilies
- 1 cup water
- 2 tablespoon soy sauce
- 2 lb. mussels

DIRECTIONS

1. Place all ingredients in a pot and bring to a boil
2. Simmer on medium heat for 12-15 minutes
3. Cover with a lid and cook until mussels cover up
4. Serve when ready

Serves: **4**

Prep Time: **10**   Minutes

Cook Time: **20**   Minutes

Total Time: **30**   Minutes

INGREDIENTS

- 2 tsp Chile powder
- 2 tsp salt
- 1 tsp cumin
- 1 tsp onion powder
- 2 tablespoons lime juice
- 2 lb. shrimp
- 1 green pepper
- 1 red onion

DIRECTIONS

1. **Mix all spices together and place fajita aside**
2. **Toss the shrimp with fajita seasoning and let marinate for a couple of minutes**

3. In a skillet heat oil and cook shrimp until soft
4. When ready remove from the skillet and serve

Serves: *2*
Prep Time: *10* Minutes

Cook Time: *20* Minutes

Total Time: *30* Minutes

INGREDIENTS

- 1 cup water
- 2 tablespoons lemon juice
- 2 garlic cloves
- 1 tsp thyme
- 1 lb. clams
- ¼ tsp salt

DIRECTIONS

1. In a skillet heat olive oil and sauté garlic, onion and thyme for 4-5 minutes
2. Add water, salt, lemon juice and clams
3. Cover with a lid and cook until shells open up
4. Serve when ready

Serves: **6-8**

Prep Time: **10**   Minutes

Cook Time: **5**   Hours

Total Time: **5**   Hours 10 Minutes

INGREDIENTS

- 1 chicken
- 1 tsp paprika
- 1 tsp salt
- 1 tsp pepper
- 1 tsp garlic powder
- 1 tsp basil
- 1 tsp oregano
- 4-5 lemon slices
- 4-5 potato slices

DIRECTIONS

1. **Mix all spices together and rub the chicken with the mixture**

2. Stuff the chicken with lemon and potato slices

3. Place the chicken into the slow cooker and cook on medium for 4-5 hours

4. When ready remove from the slow cooker and serve

Serves: **2**
Prep Time: **5**   Minutes

Cook Time: **5**   Minutes

Total Time: **10**   Minutes

INGREDIENTS

- 1 cup broccoli
- 1 cup quinoa
- 2 radishes
- 2 tablespoons pumpkin seeds
- 1 cup salad dressing

DIRECTIONS

1. In a bowl mix all ingredients and mix well
2. Serve with dressing

Serves: 2
Prep Time: 5   Minutes

Cook Time: 5   Minutes

Total Time: 10   Minutes

INGREDIENTS

- ¼ cup walnuts
- 2 radicchios
- 2 peaches
- ¼ cup parsley
- 2 scallions
- ¼ cup olive oil

DIRECTIONS

1. In a bowl mix all ingredients and mix well
2. Serve with dressing

Serves: **2**

Prep Time: **5**   Minutes

Cook Time: **5**   Minutes

Total Time: **10**   Minutes

INGREDIENTS

- 2 tablespoons lime juice
- 1 tsp hot sauce
- 2 cups grilled corn
- 2 tablespoons butter
- 2 scallions

DIRECTIONS

1. **In a bowl mix all ingredients and mix well**
2. **Serve with dressing**

Serves: **2**
Prep Time: **5**   Minutes

Cook Time: **5**   Minutes

Total Time: **10**   Minutes

INGREDIENTS

- 1 cup cherry tomatoes
- 3 tablespoons olive oil
- 1 lb. tomato slices
- 6 oz. mozzarella cheese
- Basil leaves

DIRECTIONS

1. In a bowl mix all ingredients and mix well
2. Serve with dressing

Serves: *2*
Prep Time: *5*   Minutes

Cook Time: *5*   Minutes

Total Time: *10* Minutes

INGREDIENTS

- 1 shallot
- 1 tsp lemon juice
- 1 tablespoon red wine vinegar
- 6 oz. snap peas
- 1 bunch radishes
- 2 cucumbers
- 1 romaine heart
- 4 oz. feta cheese
- 1 cup dill

DIRECTIONS

1. In a bowl mix all ingredients and mix well
2. Serve with dressing

Serves: 2
Prep Time: 5   Minutes

Cook Time: 5   Minutes

Total Time: *10*   Minutes

INGREDIENTS

- 1 jicama
- 1 mango
- ¼ cup lime juice
- 1 honeydew
- Seasoning

DIRECTIONS

1. In a bowl mix all ingredients and mix well
2. Serve with dressing

Serves: **2**

Prep Time: **5** Minutes

Cook Time: **5** Minutes

Total Time: **10** Minutes

INGREDIENTS

- 1 cup farro
- 1 shallot
- 1 tablespoon mint
- 1 lemon
- 2 cups arugula
- 1 cup baby spinach
- 1 cup mizuna
- 2 boiled eggs

DIRECTIONS

1. In a bowl mix all ingredients and mix well
2. Serve with dressing

Serves: **2**
Prep Time: **5**   Minutes

Cook Time: **5**   Minutes

Total Time: **10**   Minutes

INGREDIENTS

- 2 cucumbers
- 1 tablespoon lemon juice
- 1 celery stick
- 2 tablespoons olive oil

DIRECTIONS

1. In a bowl mix all ingredients and mix well
2. Serve with dressing

Serves: *2*

Prep Time: *5*   Minutes

Cook Time: *5*   Minutes

Total Time: *10*   Minutes

INGREDIENTS

- 2 bacon slices
- 1 tablespoon tahini sauce
- 1 tablespoon fish sauce
- 2 tablespoons lemon juice
- 2 hard boiled eggs
- 2 cooked chicken breasts
- 1 green leaf lettuce
- 2 scallions

DIRECTIONS

1. In a bowl mix all ingredients and mix well
2. Serve with dressing

WATERCRESS SALAD

Serves: **2**
Prep Time: **5**   Minutes

Cook Time: **5**   Minutes

Total Time: **10** Minutes

INGREDIENTS

- 2 tsp fish sauce
- 1 tsp hot sauce
- 1 lb. rib eye
- 1 tablespoon lemon juice
- 1 tablespoon olive oil
- 1 bunch watercress
- 2 cucumbers

DIRECTIONS

1. In a bowl mix all ingredients and mix well
2. Serve with dressing

CAULIFLOWER RECIPE

Serves: *6-8*
Prep Time: *10*   Minutes

Cook Time: *15*   Minutes

Total Time: *25*   Minutes

INGREDIENTS

- 1 pizza crust
- ½ cup tomato sauce
- ¼ black pepper
- 1 cup cauliflower
- 1 cup mozzarella cheese
- 1 cup olives

DIRECTIONS

1. Spread tomato sauce on the pizza crust
2. Place all the toppings on the pizza crust
3. Bake the pizza at 425 F for 12-15 minutes

4. When ready remove pizza from the oven and serve

Serves: **6-8**
Prep Time: **10**   Minutes

Cook Time: **15**   Minutes

Total Time: **25**   Minutes

INGREDIENTS

- 1 pizza crust
- ½ cup tomato sauce
- ¼ black pepper
- 1 cup broccoli
- 1 cup mozzarella cheese
- 1 cup olives

DIRECTIONS

1. Spread tomato sauce on the pizza crust
2. Place all the toppings on the pizza crust
3. Bake the pizza at 425 F for 12-15 minutes
4. When ready remove pizza from the oven and serve

Serves: *6-8*
Prep Time: *10*   Minutes

Cook Time: *15*   Minutes

Total Time: *25*   Minutes

INGREDIENTS

- 1 pizza crust
- ½ cup tomato sauce
- ¼ black pepper
- 1 cup pepperoni slices
- 1 cup tomatoes
- 6-8 ham slices
- 1 cup mozzarella cheese
- 1 cup olives

DIRECTIONS

1. Spread tomato sauce on the pizza crust
2. Place all the toppings on the pizza crust
3. Bake the pizza at 425 F for 12-15 minutes

4. When ready remove pizza from the oven and serve

Serves: **4**

Prep Time: **10** Minutes

Cook Time: **20** Minutes

Total Time: **30** Minutes

INGREDIENTS

- 1 tablespoon olive oil
- 1 lb. mushrooms
- ¼ red onion
- ½ cup all-purpose flour
- ¼ tsp salt
- ¼ tsp pepper
- 1 can vegetable broth
- 1 cup heavy cream

DIRECTIONS

1. **In a saucepan heat olive oil and sauté mushrooms until tender**
2. **Add remaining ingredients to the saucepan and bring to a boil**

3. When all the vegetables are tender transfer to a blender and blend until smooth

4. Pour soup into bowls, garnish with parsley and serve

Serves: **4**

Prep Time: **10** Minutes

Cook Time: **20** Minutes

Total Time: **30** Minutes

INGREDIENTS

- 1 tablespoon olive oil
- 1 lb. eggplant
- ¼ red onion
- ½ cup all-purpose flour
- ¼ tsp salt
- ¼ tsp pepper
- 1 can vegetable broth
- 1 cup heavy cream

DIRECTIONS

1. In a saucepan heat olive oil and sauté onion until tender
2. Add remaining ingredients to the saucepan and bring to a boil

5. When all the vegetables are tender transfer to a blender and blend until smooth

6. Pour soup into bowls, garnish with parsley and serve

Serves: *4*

Prep Time: *10*   Minutes

Cook Time: *20*   Minutes

Total Time: *30*   Minutes

INGREDIENTS

- 1 tablespoon olive oil
- 1 lb. cauliflower
- ¼ red onion
- ½ cup all-purpose flour
- ¼ tsp salt
- ¼ tsp pepper
- 1 can vegetable broth
- 1 cup heavy cream

DIRECTIONS

1. In a saucepan heat olive oil and sauté spinach until tender
2. Add remaining ingredients to the saucepan and bring to a boil

3. When all the vegetables are tender transfer to a blender and blend until smooth

4. Pour soup into bowls, garnish with parsley and serve

Serves: *4*
Prep Time: *10*   Minutes

Cook Time: *20*   Minutes

Total Time: *30*   Minutes

INGREDIENTS

- 1 tablespoon olive oil
- 1 lb. carrots
- ¼ red onion
- ½ cup all-purpose flour
- ¼ tsp salt
- ¼ tsp pepper
- 1 can vegetable broth
- 1 cup heavy cream

DIRECTIONS

1. In a saucepan heat olive oil and sauté onion until tender
2. Add remaining ingredients to the saucepan and bring to a boil

3. When all the vegetables are tender transfer to a blender and blend until smooth

4. Pour soup into bowls, garnish with parsley and serve

Serves: *4*
Prep Time: *10* Minutes

Cook Time: *20* Minutes

Total Time: *30* Minutes

INGREDIENTS

- 1 tablespoon olive oil
- 1 lb. asparagus
- ¼ red onion
- ½ cup all-purpose flour
- ¼ tsp salt
- ¼ tsp pepper
- 1 can vegetable broth
- 1 cup heavy cream

DIRECTIONS

1. In a saucepan heat olive oil and sauté onion until tender
2. Add remaining ingredients to the saucepan and bring to a boil

3. When all the vegetables are tender transfer to a blender and blend until smooth

4. Pour soup into bowls, garnish with parsley and serve

MANGO SMOOTHIE

Serves: *1*
Prep Time: *5*   Minutes

Cook Time: *5*   Minutes

Total Time: *10*   Minutes

INGREDIENTS

- 1 cup coconut milk
- 1 cup vanilla yogurt
- 1 cup ice
- 1 banana
- 1 mango
- 1 tsp vanilla
- 1 tsp honey

DIRECTIONS

1. In a blender place all ingredients and blend until smooth
2. Pour smoothie in a glass and serve

POWER SMOOTHIE

Serves: *1*
Prep Time: *5*   Minutes

Cook Time: *5*   Minutes

Total Time: *10*   Minutes

INGREDIENTS

- 2 cups blueberries
- 1 cup pomegranate juice
- 1 cup ice
- 1 tablespoon chia seeds
- 1 banana

DIRECTIONS

1. In a blender place all ingredients and blend until smooth
2. Pour smoothie in a glass and serve

Serves: *1*
Prep Time: 5 Minutes

Cook Time: 5 Minutes

Total Time: *10* Minutes

INGREDIENTS

- 1 cup orange juice
- 1 cup coconut water
- 1 banana
- 1 mango
- 2 cups spinach

DIRECTIONS

1. In a blender place all ingredients and blend until smooth
2. Pour smoothie in a glass and serve

Serves: *1*
Prep Time: 5   Minutes

Cook Time: 5   Minutes

Total Time: *10*   Minutes

INGREDIENTS

- 1 banana
- 1 cup blueberries
- 1 tsp ginger
- 2 cups kale leaves
- 1 cup coconut water
- 1 pinch cinnamon

DIRECTIONS

1. In a blender place all ingredients and blend until smooth
2. Pour smoothie in a glass and serve

Serves: **1**

Prep Time: **5**   Minutes

Cook Time: **5**   Minutes

Total Time: **10** Minutes

INGREDIENTS

- 1 banana
- 1 cup mango
- 1 cup blueberries
- 1 cup Greek Yogurt
- 1 tablespoon honey
- ¼ avocado

DIRECTIONS

1. In a blender place all ingredients and blend until smooth
2. Pour smoothie in a glass and serve

Serves: **1**

Prep Time: **5** Minutes

Cook Time: **5** Minutes

Total Time: **10** Minutes

INGREDIENTS

- ¼ cup oats
- 1 cup almond milk
- 1 cup cranberry juice
- ¼ cup orange juice
- 1 tablespoon honey
- 1 pinch cinnamon

DIRECTIONS

1. In a blender place all ingredients and blend until smooth
2. Pour smoothie in a glass and serve

Serves: **1**
Prep Time: **5**   Minutes

Cook Time: **5**   Minutes

Total Time: **10** Minutes

INGREDIENTS

- 1 cup coconut water
- 1 mandarin orange
- 1 cup frozen blueberries
- 1 tablespoon honey

DIRECTIONS

1. In a blender place all ingredients and blend until smooth
2. Pour smoothie in a glass and serve

Serves: **1**

Prep Time: **5**   Minutes

Cook Time: **5**   Minutes

Total Time: **10** Minutes

INGREDIENTS

- 1 banana
- ¼ cup yogurt
- 1 cup papaya
- 1 cup raspberries
- ¼ cup coconut milk
- 1 pinch cinnamon

DIRECTIONS

1. In a blender place all ingredients and blend until smooth
2. Pour smoothie in a glass and serve

PURPLE SMOOTHIE

Serves: **1**

Prep Time: **5** Minutes

Cook Time: **5** Minutes

Total Time: **10** Minutes

INGREDIENTS

- 1 cup vanilla yogurt
- 1 cup blueberries
- 1 cup blackberries
- 1 cup strawberries
- 1 banana
- 2 tablespoons honey
- 1 cup ice

DIRECTIONS

1. In a blender place all ingredients and blend until smooth
2. Pour smoothie in a glass and serve

Serves: *1*
Prep Time: 5   Minutes

Cook Time: 5   Minutes

Total Time: *10*   Minutes

INGREDIENTS

- 1 cup pineapple
- 4-5 kale leaves
- ½ cup baby spinach
- 1 cucumber
- 1 kiwi
- ½ avocado
- 1 cup ice

DIRECTIONS

1. In a blender place all ingredients and blend until smooth
2. Pour smoothie in a glass and serve

THANK YOU FOR READING THIS BOOK!

Made in the USA
Monee, IL
06 October 2020